# THE EXPECTANT MOTHER

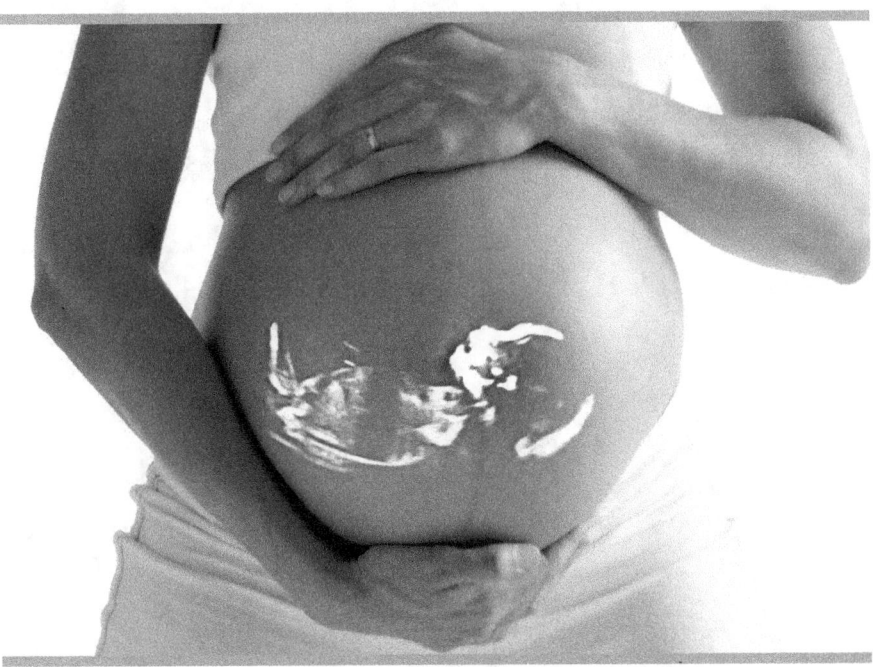

## A COMPREHENSIVE GUIDE TO A HEALTHY PREGNANCY AND CHILDBIRTH

LUCILLE J. STOKES

# COPYRIGHT

# DISCLAIMER

The information contained in this book is for general information purposes only. The author makes no representations or warranties of any kind, express or implied, about the completeness, accuracy, reliability, suitability, or availability with respect to the book or the information, products, services, or related graphics contained in the book for any purpose. Any reliance you place on such information is therefore strictly at your own risk. In no event will the author be liable for any loss or damage including without limitation, indirect or consequential loss or damage, or any loss or damage whatsoever arising from loss of data or profits arising out of, or in connection with, the use of this book.

# TABLE OF CONTENTS

# INTRODUCTION

Pregnancy and childbirth are some of the most transformative experiences a person can go through. As soon as the decision to start a family is made, it can feel like the start of an incredible journey filled with anticipation, excitement, and a hint of nervousness. Preparing for pregnancy can be intense, but it's important to remember that every step of the way is worth it.

From the first trimester, when the tiny seed of life takes root, to the second, where the bond between mother and child begins to form, and finally the third, where the anticipation of meeting the little bundle of joy peaks, every moment is a new adventure. The love and dedication that go into bringing a new life into the world are unparalleled, and the journey towards motherhood is nothing short of awe-inspiring.

Yet, along with all of the beauty and wonder of pregnancy and childbirth, come challenges and obstacles. The physical and emotional changes that happen during pregnancy can be exhausting and overwhelming. It's vital to find ways to manage them while still cherishing the joy that comes with building a new family.

Labor and delivery are, without question, the most intense and emotional moments of the journey. Every woman's experience is unique and miraculous, yet all share a common bond of strength and resilience throughout the birthing process.

Postpartum care and the occurrence of postpartum depression can also be difficult experiences, but there is help and support available for new mothers.

This book is a comprehensive guide to every aspect of pregnancy and childbirth. From special situations, to adjusting to your new family and everything in between, this book covers it all. We hope that this comprehensive guide will provide you with the knowledge, tools, and support you need to navigate this incredible journey, embrace the challenges, and cherish the joys of pregnancy and childbirth.

Here's a brief overview of what each chapter in the book about pregnancy and childbirth will cover:

Chapter 1: Preparing for Pregnancy - This chapter will provide helpful tips and advice for preparing to conceive, such as balancing hormones, healthy eating, and lifestyle changes.

Chapter 2: The First Trimester - This chapter will cover the early stages of pregnancy, from weeks 1-12, including the physical and emotional changes that occur in the mother and fetus during this time.

Chapter 3: The Second Trimester - This chapter will cover the middle stages of pregnancy, from weeks 13-27, including fetal development, common symptoms, and prenatal care.

Chapter 4: The Third Trimester - This chapter will cover the final stages of pregnancy, from weeks 28-40 (or until delivery), including fetal growth and development, preparing for labor and delivery, and coping with physical and emotional changes.

Chapter 5: Labor and Delivery - This chapter will cover the stages of labor and delivery, including common medical interventions, pain management options, and postpartum care.

Chapter 6: Postpartum Care - This chapter will provide information on the physical and emotional care required in the days and weeks following childbirth. It will cover topics like breastfeeding, postpartum depression, and returning to activities and work.

Chapter 7: Postpartum Depression - This chapter will look at postpartum depression in detail, including its causes, symptoms, and treatment options.

Chapter 8: Special Situations - This chapter will cover common challenges and complications that may arise during pregnancy and childbirth, such as high-risk pregnancies, multiple births, and preterm labor.

Chapter 9: Your New Family - This chapter will provide practical advice on adjusting to life with a newborn, including developing routines, sleep management tips, and adjusting to family dynamics.

Each chapter will be designed to inform and guide the reader with helpful tips, personal experiences, and practical advice to provide reassurance and confidence as they navigate the various stages of pregnancy and childbirth.

# CHAPTER 1

## PREPARING FOR PREGNANCY

### Factors to consider before getting pregnant

1. Health and medical history:

Health and medical history is an essential aspect of ensuring a healthy pregnancy and successful fertility. Therefore, it is crucial to discuss with a healthcare provider about any preexisting medical conditions, medications, and family medical history that could affect fertility and pregnancy. Certain medical conditions, like thyroid disorders, autoimmune diseases, genetic disorders, and sexually transmitted diseases, can adversely impact fertility. Thus, it is necessary to identify and manage such conditions before planning for pregnancy.

It is also essential to review any medications that have been prescribed by a doctor, including over-the-counter drugs, supplements, and herbal remedies. Some medications can negatively affect fertility or harm the fetus in the early stages of pregnancy. Therefore, it is crucial to confirm that the medications taken do not pose any risks to either fertility or pregnancy.

Family medical history can also play an integral role in fertility and pregnancy. Some genetic conditions passed on through generations may impact the ability to conceive or increase the risk of miscarriage or birth defects. For example, a family history of recurrent miscarriage, premature birth, or stillbirth may warrant further investigation before planning pregnancy. Therefore, discussing family medical history with a healthcare provider can help in assessing the risk factors and managing any underlying medical conditions appropriately.

Overall, taking a comprehensive medical history before pregnancy can help in identifying risks that might affect fertility and pregnancy, and appropriate measures can be taken to manage or treat any underlying medical conditions. This can contribute to a healthy pregnancy and ensure the best possible health outcomes for the mother and child.

2. Lifestyle and habits:

Lifestyle and habits significantly impact fertility and pregnancy outcomes. Certain unhealthy habits like smoking, drinking alcohol, and drug use can negatively affect fertility and increase the risk of complications during pregnancy, leading to preterm births, low birth weight, congenital disabilities, and even stillbirths. Therefore, it is advised to quit such habits before planning to conceive.

Smoking is one of the leading causes of infertility, and it can also harm the fetus during pregnancy. Studies have shown that smoking can reduce both male and female fertility and increase the risk of complications like ectopic pregnancy, miscarriage, placental complications, and preterm deliveries during pregnancy.

Alcohol consumption can also affect fertility, and excessive drinking can also increase the risk of fetal alcohol syndrome (FAS) during pregnancy. FAS is a severe condition that causes growth deficiencies and cognitive and behavioral impairments in the fetus.

Drug use, including recreational drugs or prescription drugs not approved for pregnancy, can cause negative effects on fertility and fetal development. Many drugs can harm the fetus, leading to developmental disorders, physical abnormalities, and even stillbirth.

Therefore, it is recommended to quit such habits before planning to conceive. Studies have shown that quitting smoking, alcohol, and drug use several months before conception can lead to significant improvements in fertility rates and reduce fetal harm during pregnancy. It is also essential to maintain a healthy lifestyle by eating a balanced diet, staying physically active, and getting enough rest to prepare the body for pregnancy.

In conclusion, taking care of one's lifestyle and habits can positively impact fertility and pregnancy outcomes. Quitting unhealthy habits like smoking, alcohol, and drug use is essential to ensure a healthy pregnancy and a healthy baby.

3. Nutrition:

Nutrition plays a crucial role in fertility and pregnancy outcomes. Eating a well-balanced diet with enough vitamins, minerals, and essential nutrients is important for ensuring optimal health for both the mother and the developing fetus. Therefore, it is essential to eat nutritiously and maintain a healthy weight before getting pregnant to ensure the best possible health outcomes for the baby and the mother.

A diet that is low in essential nutrients can affect fertility and increase the risk of complications during pregnancy. Women who are not getting enough calories, protein, vitamins, minerals, and other essential nutrients may experience menstrual cycle irregularities and difficulty in ovulation. Furthermore, poor nutrition during pregnancy can lead to low birth weight, preterm birth, and other complications during childbirth.

Therefore, it is recommended that women who are planning to conceive should eat a well-balanced diet that includes a variety of fruits, vegetables, whole grains, lean meats, and dairy products. It is also important to avoid foods that can be harmful to the developing fetus, such as raw or undercooked meat, certain types of fish that contain high levels of mercury, unpasteurized dairy products, and some types of soft cheeses.

Maintaining a healthy weight before pregnancy is also crucial for fertility and pregnancy outcomes. Being overweight or underweight may negatively impact fertility and increase the risk of complications during pregnancy. Therefore, it is important to work with a healthcare provider to maintain a healthy weight and incorporate regular physical activity to prepare the body for pregnancy.

In conclusion, a well-balanced diet and maintenance of a healthy weight are pivotal for optimal fertility and ensuring the best possible outcomes during pregnancy. Planning for pregnancy should be done after making significant lifestyle changes, including adopting a healthy diet, maintaining a healthy weight, and avoiding unhealthy habits. Consulting with a healthcare provider can provide guidance on making these lifestyle changes to enhance your health and the health of your future baby.

4. Mental and emotional health:

Mental and emotional health is crucial for a successful pregnancy and healthy birth outcomes. Pregnancy can be a stressful time that comes with many physical and emotional changes, so taking steps to manage stress, anxiety, depression, and other mental health issues before trying to conceive is essential.

Stress, anxiety, and depression can negatively impact fertility and increase the likelihood of complications during pregnancy. Research has shown that high levels of stress and anxiety can affect ovulation and fertility in women and sperm quality and motility in men. Depression during pregnancy can also increase the risk of preterm birth, low birth weight, and other complications.

Therefore, taking care of your mental and emotional health before conception is important. It's recommended to seek help if you are experiencing symptoms of depression, anxiety, or other mental health issues. This may include talking to a healthcare provider or mental health professional, practicing relaxation techniques, getting enough sleep, and engaging in physical activity.

It may also be beneficial to establish a support system of family and friends to help manage stress during pregnancy. Building a support system can provide emotional support, help with daily tasks, and reduce feelings of isolation and loneliness during pregnancy.

In conclusion, mental and emotional health is a vital aspect of fertility and pregnancy outcomes. Taking steps to manage stress, anxiety, depression, and other mental health issues before conceiving can improve fertility rates and reduce the risk of complications during pregnancy. Remember to seek support from healthcare providers, family and friends, and professionals to ensure optimal mental and emotional health during pregnancy.

5. Finances:

Planning for the financial costs associated with pregnancy, childbirth, and raising a child is an important consideration for couples who are planning to have a baby. Having a child can be a significant financial commitment, so it's important to plan ahead and ensure that you are financially prepared.

There are many financial costs associated with pregnancy, such as medical expenses, including prenatal care, ultrasounds, and childbirth classes, as well as the cost of childbirth itself. After the baby is born, there are also costs associated with childcare, such as diapers, formula, baby gear, and daycare expenses. Additionally, there are long-term costs associated with raising a child, such as education and healthcare costs.

Therefore, it is important to consider the financial aspects of having a child before getting pregnant. Couples can start by creating a budget to determine their current expenses and identify areas where they can cut back to save money. It is also important to research the cost of medical care and other expenses associated with pregnancy and childbirth. Health insurance plans, maternity and paternity leave, and potential childcare expenses should be considered as part of financial planning.

Another important consideration is building an emergency fund in case of unexpected expenses related to pregnancy or childbirth. It's also important to have a plan for income during the period of time that either parent may need to take off work for the birth of the child.

In conclusion, planning for the financial costs that come with pregnancy, childbirth, and raising a child, should be a priority when deciding to have a baby. Couples can start by creating a budget, researching the costs of medical care and other expenses associated with having a child, building an emergency fund, and having a plan for income during absences from work. By taking these steps, couples can ensure that they are financially prepared to start a family and provide the best for their child's future.

6. Support system:

Building and maintaining a strong support system is important for expectant parents during pregnancy. A supportive partner, family, and friends can help alleviate stress, offer encouragement, and provide practical assistance during this exciting and challenging time.

A supportive partner is particularly important as they can provide emotional support, help with daily tasks, and attend doctor appointments. It is also important to communicate with your partner about your expectations and needs during pregnancy to ensure that sharing caregiving responsibilities is part of your support system.

Expectant parents can also build a supportive network with family and friends who can help in practical ways such as providing transportation, preparing meals, and helping with household chores and baby gear setup. Friends who have recently gone through pregnancy and childbirth can offer advice, recommendations, and a listening ear.

Other supportive resources include prenatal classes, pregnancy support groups, and healthcare providers who can offer guidance and emotional support throughout pregnancy.

Maintaining a strong support system after the baby is born is also essential as the first few months of a baby's life can be overwhelming for new parents. Family and friends can continue to offer practical assistance, provide childcare, and offer emotional support to alleviate stress during this transition.

In conclusion, building and maintaining a strong support system is important for expectant parents during pregnancy. A supportive partner, family, and friends can provide encouragement and practical assistance that can make the pregnancy journey easier. It is essential to communicate your needs and expectations with your support system to ensure that everyone is on the same page during this exciting time.

7. Age:

Age is an important factor to consider when planning for pregnancy. Fertility declines as women age, which can make it more difficult to conceive. Therefore, considering the best age for conceiving based on individual circumstances is important for couples who are planning to have a baby.

Women generally have their highest fertility in their 20s and early 30s, after which their fertility begins to decline. By age 35, the decline in fertility becomes steeper. This means that women who delay pregnancy until later in life may have a harder time getting pregnant and may need to consider fertility treatments to conceive.

However, age is not the only factor that affects fertility. Other factors such as overall health, family history, and lifestyle choices, such as smoking and alcohol consumption, can also impact fertility.

Women who are older or have a history of fertility problems may want to consider seeking the advice of a fertility specialist before trying to conceive. Fertility treatments such as in vitro fertilization (IVF) and egg freezing may be options for women who are having difficulty conceiving.

It's important to note that while age can affect fertility, it is not impossible to conceive at an older age. Couples should consider their personal circumstances and consult with a healthcare provider to make an informed decision about the best age for them to conceive.

In conclusion, age is an important factor to consider when planning for pregnancy. Couples should be aware of the decline in fertility as women age and consider seeking the advice of a fertility specialist if needed. However, it's important to note that age is not the only factor that affects fertility, and couples should make an informed decision based on their individual circumstances.

8. Work and career:

Work and career choices can certainly affect pregnancy decisions and outcomes. Expectant parents need to consider the impact their jobs may have on pregnancy, childbirth, and caring for a new baby.

One important consideration is maternity leave. It is important for expectant mothers to know their company's maternity leave policy and plan accordingly. Many companies offer paid maternity leave, while others offer only unpaid leave or no maternity leave at all. Women who are self-employed or working in jobs without paid leave may need to plan for income loss during their time off.

It's important to note that in the United States, the Family and Medical Leave Act (FMLA) provides up to 12 weeks of unpaid leave for eligible employees to care for a new child. However, this does not guarantee paid leave, and not all employees are eligible, so it's important to know your rights under the law.

Another important consideration is workplace support. Pregnant women and new parents may need additional support from their employers, coworkers, and/or human resources department. This may include accommodations for physical limitations or doctor's appointments, flexible work arrangements (such as telecommuting or reduced hours), and lactation support.

It is also important to consider the safety of the job environment as some jobs may be more physically demanding or have exposure to harmful substances that can potentially harm a developing fetus.

In conclusion, work and career choices can have a significant impact on pregnancy decisions and outcomes. Expectant parents should consider their company's maternity leave policy, plan for income loss during leave if needed, and seek support from their workplace. Additionally, they should keep in mind any safety concerns or limitations in order to protect themselves and their unborn child.

## Preconception Health: Increasing the Chances of Conception

Preconception health refers to the health of individuals before they try to conceive a baby. It is an important aspect of pregnancy planning and can impact the health of the mother and the baby. In this article, we will discuss the key aspects of preconception health and how to increase the chances of conception.

1. Get a Preconception Checkup: A preconception checkup is an important step in ensuring good health before pregnancy.

During this checkup, healthcare providers will review medical history, medications, vaccinations, and lifestyle factors such as nutrition, exercise, and substance use. It's important to address any health concerns or underlying conditions before pregnancy, as they can impact pregnancy outcomes.

2. Maintain a Healthy Diet: A well-balanced diet that is high in fruits, vegetables, whole grains, and lean proteins is key to maintaining good health. In addition, taking folic acid supplements can help prevent neural tube defects in the baby. The recommended daily amount of folic acid is 400 to 800 micrograms per day, and it is recommended to start taking folic acid supplements at least one month before trying to conceive.

3. Exercise Regularly: Regular exercise is important for overall health, and can help increase fertility by regulating menstrual cycles and improving ovulation. Moderate exercises such as brisk walking, swimming, and cycling are all safe during preconception and pregnancy. However, it is important to consult with a healthcare provider before starting any new exercise regimen.

4. Manage Stress: Stress can have a negative impact on fertility and pregnancy outcomes. It's important to manage stress levels through techniques such as meditation, yoga, or counseling. Consistent exercise and a healthy diet can also help reduce stress levels.

5. Avoid Harmful Substances: Smoking, alcohol, and recreational drug use can all decrease fertility and increase the risk of birth defects. It is recommended to quit smoking and avoid alcohol and illicit drugs before conception.

6. Maintain a Healthy Weight: Being overweight or underweight can affect fertility and increase the risk of pregnancy complications. Staying within a healthy weight range by maintaining a healthy diet and exercising regularly can increase the chances of conception.

7. Monitor Ovulation: Monitoring ovulation can help identify the most fertile days of the menstrual cycle and increase the chances of conception. This can be done through at-home ovulation predictor kits or monitoring basal body temperature.

In conclusion, preconception health is an important aspect of pregnancy planning. Maintaining a healthy lifestyle by eating a healthy diet, getting regular exercise, managing stress, avoiding harmful substances, maintaining a healthy weight, and monitoring ovulation can all increase the chances of conception and promote a healthy pregnancy.

# CHAPTER 2

## THE FIRST TRIMESTER

### Physical and emotional changes during the first trimester

The first trimester of pregnancy is a time of significant physical and emotional changes as the body undergoes many adjustments to support the growing fetus. In this article, we will discuss the typical physical and emotional changes that occur during the first trimester of pregnancy.

Physical Changes:

1. Morning Sickness: Many women experience nausea and vomiting during the first trimester, typically peaking at around 9 weeks. This condition is often referred to as "morning sickness," but it can occur at any time of the day.

2. Fatigue: It is common for women to experience fatigue

during the first trimester due to the increase in the hormone progesterone, which can cause drowsiness.

3. Breast Changes: The breasts may become sore, swollen, and/or tender as the body prepares for lactation.

4. Frequent Urination: As the uterus expands, it puts pressure on the bladder, causing women to need to urinate more frequently.

5. Cravings and Aversions: Many women experience food cravings and aversions during the first trimester, which can be influenced by hormonal changes and increased sensitivity to smell.

Emotional Changes:

1. Mood Swings: Hormonal changes can cause mood swings, irritability, and emotional sensitivity during the first trimester.

2. Anxiety: Many women experience anxiety and worry about the health and well-being of the growing fetus, as well as concerns about the upcoming changes to their lifestyle.

3. Excitement: Despite the physical discomfort and emotional changes, many women feel excited and happy about the pregnancy, particularly as they start to see the first signs of

the baby's growth.

4. Fear of Miscarriage: The risk of miscarriage is highest during the first trimester, which can cause significant anxiety and stress for women.

5. Changes in Relationships: Pregnancy can cause changes in personal and professional relationships, as women may need to adjust their lifestyle to accommodate the pregnancy.

The first trimester of pregnancy is a time of significant physical and emotional changes. Women may experience nausea, fatigue, breast changes, frequent urination, and food cravings or aversions. They may also experience mood swings, anxiety, excitement, fear of miscarriage, and changes in relationships. These changes are a normal part of pregnancy, but it's important to speak with a healthcare provider if they become overwhelming or interfere with daily life.

## How to deal with morning sickness and other pregnancy-related symptoms

Pregnancy can be an exciting time, but the physical and emotional changes can also be challenging. Morning sickness, fatigue, and other symptoms can make it difficult to enjoy the experience. In this article, we will discuss some tips for dealing with common pregnancy-related symptoms.

1. Morning Sickness: Morning sickness is a common symptom experienced by many pregnant women during the first trimester, although it can sometimes extend throughout pregnancy. Nausea and vomiting can be challenging and affect daily activities. While there are some medications that may offer relief, many women prefer to use natural remedies to help manage their symptoms.

Morning sickness can be a challenging symptom to deal with, but there are natural remedies that women may find helpful. Ginger, peppermint, chamomile, vitamin B6, and other home remedies may provide relief for some women. It is essential to speak with a healthcare provider before trying any new supplements or herbs and to take steps to care for yourself and your growing baby.

The following are tips for you to deal with morning sickness:

Other home remedies for morning sickness include:

Eating small, frequent meals throughout the day, rather than three large meals

- Avoiding foods or smells that trigger nausea

- Staying hydrated by drinking plenty of water

- Eating protein-rich foods and complex carbohydrates

- Getting enough rest and taking naps when needed

- Practicing relaxation techniques, such as deep breathing and gentle exercise.

Herbal remedies have also been used at home to reduce the effect of morning sickness.

One herbal remedy that can provide relief for morning sickness is ginger. Ginger root contains compounds that help settle the stomach and reduce inflammation. It can be taken in various forms, including fresh or dried ginger, ginger tea, or ginger capsules. Some studies even suggest that ginger may be as effective as over-the-counter medications in reducing nausea and vomiting.

Other herbs and supplements that may provide relief for morning sickness include peppermint, chamomile, and vitamin B6. Peppermint tea may help soothe nausea, and chamomile tea can provide a calming effect. Vitamin B6 supplements, at a dosage of up to 25mg, are recommended, since it has antiemetic efficacy without side effects when taken orally throughout the day.

It is essential to talk to a healthcare provider before using any natural remedies or supplements during pregnancy. While many herbs and supplements are generally considered safe, their effects on pregnancy can vary. Additionally, certain natural remedies can interact with medications or have side effects, so it is essential to discuss their use with a healthcare provider.

2. Fatigue: It's common to feel tired during pregnancy, particularly during the first trimester. Getting adequate rest, eating a healthy, balanced diet, and moderate exercise can help manage fatigue.

3. Constipation: Constipation is a common symptom of pregnancy due to hormone changes and pressure from the growing uterus. To manage constipation, eat a high-fiber diet, stay hydrated, and talk to your healthcare provider about using a stool softener.

4. Back Pain: As the uterus expands, it can cause back pain. Use proper posture and gentle exercise to manage back pain. Swimming, prenatal yoga, and guided meditation can also help alleviate discomfort.

5. Heartburn: Heartburn is common during pregnancy as the growing fetus puts pressure on the stomach and acid reflux increases. Eating smaller meals throughout the day and avoiding spicy, greasy, or acidic foods can help manage

heartburn.

6. Swelling: Some women experience swelling in their feet and ankles during pregnancy due to increased blood volume. To manage swelling, avoid standing or sitting for long periods, elevate feet when sitting, and wear supportive shoes.

7. Mood Swings: Hormonal changes can cause mood swings during pregnancy. Seeking support from friends, family, or a therapist, practicing relaxation techniques, and engaging in light exercise can help manage mood swings.

Pregnancy can be challenging, but there are many strategies that can be used to manage common pregnancy symptoms. It's important to speak with healthcare providers about any persistent or severe symptoms and to take steps to care for yourself and your growing baby.

# Prenatal care and the importance of regular check-ups

Prenatal care, which involves regular medical check-ups throughout pregnancy, is essential for the health and well-being of both the mother and the developing baby. During the first trimester, regular check-ups are particularly important as it is the most critical time of fetal development.

Here are some reasons why regular check-ups during the first trimester are so important:

1. Confirm Pregnancy: The first prenatal visit is typically scheduled around 8 weeks after the last menstrual period. This visit involves a physical exam and may include an ultrasound to confirm pregnancy.

2. Monitor Fetal Development: During the first trimester, the baby's organs and tissues develop. Regular prenatal visits allow healthcare providers to monitor fetal growth and ensure that everything is progressing appropriately.

3. Screen for Health Conditions: Prenatal care includes a series of tests and screenings to check for any underlying health conditions or risk factors that could affect the pregnancy. These tests may include blood work, urine tests, and a pap

smear to test for sexually transmitted infections.

4. Manage Pregnancy Symptoms: The first trimester is when many women experience morning sickness, headaches, and other pregnancy symptoms. Healthcare providers can provide guidance and medication if necessary to manage these symptoms.

5. Provide Education: Prenatal visits provide an opportunity to discuss any questions or concerns with healthcare providers. They can also offer education on creating a healthy pregnancy, including proper nutrition, exercise, and self-care practices.

Prenatal care is critical for ensuring a healthy pregnancy and a healthy baby. Regular check-ups during the first trimester are vital for monitoring fetal development, managing pregnancy symptoms, and identifying any health conditions or risk factors that require attention. Women should schedule prenatal visits with a healthcare provider as soon as they know they are pregnant, and maintain regular check-ups throughout their pregnancy.

## Diet and nutrition

Proper nutrition is crucial during all stages of pregnancy, but it is particularly important during the first trimester. A healthy and balanced diet during the first trimester can help support fetal development, reduce the risk of birth defects, and promote overall maternal health.

Here are some essential nutrients that should be included in a healthy diet during the first trimester of pregnancy:

1. Folic Acid: Folic acid is a B vitamin that is essential for fetal development. It can help prevent birth defects of the brain and spine. Good sources of folic acid include leafy green vegetables, fortified cereals, and citrus fruits.

2. Iron: Iron is needed to make hemoglobin, the protein in red blood cells that carries oxygen throughout the body. During pregnancy, the body needs more iron to support the growing fetus. Good sources of iron include lean meats, poultry, fish, beans, and fortified cereals.

3. Protein: Protein is essential for fetal growth and development. Good sources of protein include lean meats, poultry, fish, eggs, beans, and nuts.

4. Calcium: Calcium is needed to support fetal bone development and maintain maternal bone health. Good sources of calcium include milk, cheese, yogurt, tofu, and leafy green vegetables.

5. Vitamins and Minerals: In addition to folic acid, iron, protein, and calcium, a healthy diet during the first trimester should also include a variety of vitamins and minerals, such as vitamin D, vitamin C, vitamin B6, and magnesium. Good sources of these nutrients can be found in fruits, vegetables, whole grains, and fortified cereals.

It is important to avoid some foods and drinks that can be harmful during pregnancy, such as alcohol, caffeine, and certain types of fish, including those with high levels of mercury. Additionally, pregnant women should be cautious of foodborne illnesses, such as listeria and salmonella, by avoiding certain foods, such as raw or undercooked meats, unpasteurized dairy products, and deli meats.

A healthy and balanced diet during the first trimester of pregnancy is essential for fetal development and maternal health. Foods rich in folic acid, iron, protein, calcium, vitamins, and, minerals should be included while avoiding certain foods and drinks that can be harmful. Pregnant women should speak with a healthcare provider or a registered dietitian to ensure they are getting proper nutrition during this critical time.

# CHAPTER 3

## THE SECOND TRIMESTER

The second trimester is often considered the most comfortable stage of pregnancy, as many of the unpleasant symptoms of the first trimester have subsided. However, there are still physical and emotional issues that the mother may experience during this period of pregnancy. Here are some of the common issues that pregnant women may experience during the second trimester:

## Physical Issues:

1. Growing Belly: The mother's belly will continue to grow during the second trimester, which can cause discomfort and back pain.

2. Stretch Marks: As the belly expands, the mother may develop stretch marks on her abdomen, hips, and thighs.

3. Braxton Hicks Contractions: These are mild contractions that prepare the mother's body for labor. They usually start in the second trimester.

4. Increased Energy: Many women feel more energetic during the second trimester as the fatigue of the first trimester subsides.

5. Increased Appetite: As the baby grows, the mother's appetite may increase to meet the demands of her growing baby.

## Emotional Issues:

1. Anxiety: As the due date approaches, some pregnant women experience anxiety about labor and becoming a mother.

2. Mood Swings: Hormonal changes and stress can cause mood swings in pregnant women.

3. Body Image: As her body changes, a pregnant woman may feel self-conscious about her appearance, which can affect her self-esteem.

4. Bonding with the Baby: Some women may have difficulty

feeling a strong bond with their baby before birth.

5. Sleep Disturbances: As the belly grows and other pregnancy symptoms, such as heartburn and leg cramps, can cause sleep disturbances.

The second trimester comes with its own set of physical and emotional issues. Physical symptoms such as a growing belly and stretch marks, as well as anxieties related to labor, body image concerns, and sleep disturbances, are just some of the many issues a pregnant woman might face. It's important to address these issues with a healthcare provider and to practice good self-care to ensure a healthy pregnancy and to prepare for childbirth.

Prenatal screening tests and ultrasounds

During the second trimester of pregnancy, there are several prenatal screening tests and ultrasounds that pregnant women can undergo to check on the health and development of their baby. Here are some of the tests and ultrasounds that may be recommended during the second trimester:

1. Maternal Blood Tests: Blood tests may be done during the second trimester to screen for certain chromosomal abnormalities, such as Down's syndrome. The test looks for certain proteins and hormones in the mother's blood that can

indicate a higher risk of certain genetic conditions.

2. Quad Screen or Serum Integrated Test: This is a combination of blood tests, which are usually done between 15 and 20 weeks of pregnancy. It helps detect the risks of Down syndrome, trisomy 18, and neural tube defects.

3. Ultrasound: During the second trimester, an ultrasound can detect any structural abnormalities in the baby and is typically performed around 20 weeks of pregnancy. The ultrasound can give the parents an opportunity to see the baby's physical features, sex and help evaluate fetal growth.

4. Amniocentesis: This test is offered if there is a higher risk of chromosome abnormalities or genetic disorders. During an amniocentesis, a small needle is inserted into the uterus and a small amount of amniotic fluid is removed. This fluid is then tested for genetic abnormalities.

5. Glucose Screening Test: This test is done between 24-28 weeks to check for gestational diabetes (diabetes that develops during pregnancy).

It is important to note that not all women will undergo the same tests and ultrasounds, as their medical history and personal circumstances may influence the need for certain tests. Pregnant women should talk to their healthcare provider about their individual prenatal testing plans.

## Preparing for labor and delivery

Preparing for labor and delivery can help expectant mothers feel more confident and prepared for the process. Here are some tips to prepare for labor and delivery:

1. Attend Childbirth Preparation Classes: Many hospitals or birthing centers offer childbirth preparation courses where expectant mothers and their partners can learn about the signs of labor, pain management techniques, breastfeeding, and newborn care. These classes can also provide an opportunity to ask questions and meet other expecting parents.

2. Choose a Birth Plan: A birth plan is a document that outlines the mother's preferences for labor and delivery, such as pain management, delivery positions, and whether to use medical interventions such as epidurals or forceps. Discussing the plan with the healthcare provider and making sure the hospital staff is aware of the plan can help ensure that everyone is on the same page.

3. Stay Active: Exercise during pregnancy can be beneficial for both the mother and baby and can help prepare the body

for labor and delivery. Activities such as walking, swimming, and prenatal yoga can help.

4. Practice Relaxation Techniques: Stress and anxiety can make labor and delivery more difficult, so practicing relaxation techniques such as deep breathing exercises, visualization, or taking hot baths may benefit expecting mothers.

5. Pack a Hospital Bag: Preparing a hospital bag with essentials such as comfortable clothing, toiletries, a camera, and insurance information can help ease the stress of going to the hospital for labor.

6. Discuss Pain Management Options: It is important to discuss pain management options with the healthcare provider in advance of labor and delivery. This includes natural methods such as breathing and relaxation techniques, as well as medical interventions like epidurals.

7. Create a Support System: Having a supportive partner, family member, or friend at the labor and delivery can help alleviate stress and provide emotional support during the process.

Remember, every birth experience is unique, and it is important to be flexible and prepared for unexpected changes. It is recommended to work closely with your healthcare provider and ask any questions you may have to help ensure that you are prepared for labor and delivery.

# CHAPTER 4

## THE THIRD TRIMESTER

### Changes in baby's development

A lot of changes happen to a baby during the time he or she spends in the womb. Here are some of the significant developments that occur in the baby during different trimesters:

First Trimester:

- Formation of major organs: During the first trimester, the baby's major organs, such as the heart, brain, lungs, and liver, begin to form. By the end of the first trimester, these organs are fully functional.

- Limb development: The baby's arms and legs begin to form during the first trimester, along with fingers and toes.

- Heartbeat: By around six weeks, the baby's heartbeat can usually be detected by ultrasound.

Second Trimester:

- Fetal movement: By the end of the second trimester, the baby begins to move around in the womb.

- Development of senses: The baby's senses begin to develop during the second trimester. He or she can start to hear, see, and taste.

- Growth: The baby will grow significantly during the second trimester, from around 3 inches to around 14 inches in length.

**Third Trimester:**

- Final preparations: During the third trimester, the baby prepares for life outside the womb. He or she will practice breathing, swallowing, and urinating.

- Putting on weight: The baby will put on a significant

amount of weight during the third trimester, as much as one pound per week.

- Positioning: In preparation for birth, the baby may move into a head-down position. By the end of the third trimester, most babies are in this position.

During each trimester of pregnancy, a baby develops and changes significantly as the organs and body systems form and mature. These changes help to prepare the baby for life outside of the womb. Pregnant women can monitor these changes by regularly visiting their doctors and undergoing ultrasounds.

## The role of the obstetrician and the midwife

The third trimester is a crucial period of pregnancy, and both obstetricians and midwives play an essential role in ensuring the mother and baby are healthy and safe. Here are some ways in which obstetricians and midwives contribute during the third trimester:

**Obstetricians:**

1. Check Fetal Growth: Obstetricians routinely check the baby's

growth during the third trimester to ensure that the baby is growing at a healthy rate. This often involves measuring the size of the uterus or performing an ultrasound.

2. Monitor Mom's health: The obstetrician will also monitor the mother's health and check for any signs of complications such as gestational diabetes, hypertension, preeclampsia or signs of preterm labor.

3. Prepare for Delivery: The obstetrician will work with the mother to discuss pain management options, determine if a vaginal birth or c-section is necessary, and create a delivery plan based on the health of the mother and baby.

4. Perform Tests: The obstetrician will perform important tests during the third trimester, including a Group B strep test (a bacterial infection of the genital tract), and may conduct tests to determine the fetal position or check the cervix's dilation and effacement.

**Midwives:**

1. Provide Support: Midwives provide supportive care to expectant mothers during the third trimester. They provide emotional support, answer questions about pregnancy and childbirth, and ensure that mothers feel confident and prepared for delivery.

2. Prepare for Labor: Midwives often work with mothers to create a birth plan that outlines their preferences for delivery, including natural pain management techniques, and make informed decisions during the labor and delivery process.

3. Monitor the Labor Process: Midwives play a critical role during labor and delivery. They monitor fetal heart rate, help the mother with breathing and relaxation techniques, and provide guidance on pushing.

4. Promote Breastfeeding: Midwives provide support for mothers who choose to breastfeed their babies. They help promote breastfeeding education and assist with latch-on techniques and any breastfeeding challenges.

Both obstetricians and midwives work together to support pregnant women during the third trimester, ensuring that mothers are adequately monitored and supported, and providing the care necessary for a healthy pregnancy and safe delivery.

## Physical and emotional changes during the third trimester

The third trimester of pregnancy is the final stage before the baby is delivered and is characterized by several physical and emotional changes. Here are some of the changes women may experience during this period:

**Physical Changes:**

1. Fetal Growth: The baby continues to grow rapidly during the third trimester, with the average fetal weight being around 6-8 pounds.

2. Difficulty in Breathing: As the baby grows, it may put pressure on the mother's diaphragm, making it hard for her to breathe normally.

3. Backaches and Leg Cramps: The additional weight and strain on the mother's muscles and joints can result in back pain and leg cramps.

4. Frequent Urination: The growing fetus can put pressure on the mother's bladder, leading to more frequent urination.

5. Braxton Hicks Contractions: Women may also experience Braxton Hicks or practice contractions during the third trimester. These are sporadic contractions that help prepare the uterus for labor.

**Emotional Changes:**

1. Anxiety: The soon-to-be mother may experience anxiety as the due date approaches. The anxiety may be related to concerns about delivery and the well-being of the baby.

2. Fatigue: As the mother's uterus grows bigger, it may become difficult for her to get enough sleep, leading to persistent fatigue.

3. Restlessness: Hormonal changes in the body as the due date approaches may cause restlessness and difficulty sleeping.

4. Excitement: The mother may feel excited as the due date approaches and she prepares to meet her newborn baby.

5. Nesting Instincts: Feeling the urge to organize and prepare the home for the baby's arrival is common during the third trimester.

Overall, the third trimester of pregnancy can be both physically and emotionally challenging; however, understanding the changes and coping mechanisms can help mothers-to-be manage these changes and prepare for the arrival of their baby.

# What to expect during labor and delivery

Labor and delivery can happen differently for every woman, but here are some general things to expect during this process:

1. Early Labor: The cervix starts to dilate, and contractions become stronger, longer, and more frequent. Women may experience lower back pain, cramping, and other symptoms such as diarrhea or nausea.

2. Active Labor: The cervix continues to dilate, and contractions become even stronger and more intense. This is when women start to feel pressure on their pelvis and may experience a rupture of the amniotic sac.

3. Transition: The final phase of labor, where the cervix fully dilates, and contractions become more intense, and faster.

4. Pushing: When the baby's head is visible, women will begin pushing to help deliver the baby.

5. Delivery: The baby is born as the women continue to push, and the doctor or midwife will guide the head and shoulders out while cutting the umbilical cord.

6. Placenta Delivery: After the baby is born, the uterus

continues to contract, resulting in the delivery of the placenta.

7. Recovery: Women will be monitored for hemorrhaging and other complications and pressed for skin-to-skin contact with the newborn baby within an hour of delivery.

Pain management options are also available for women during labor, including epidurals, nitrous oxide, or natural pain relief techniques such as breathing and relaxation techniques.

It's also essential to note that labor and delivery can take anywhere from several hours to a few days, and each woman's experience is unique. Women should talk to their healthcare provider about any concerns they have and have support available throughout the process.

## Birthing options - natural birth vs. epidurals

Natural birth and epidurals are popular birthing options available to women during labor and delivery. Here are some detailed discussions on both birthing options:

Natural Birth:

Natural childbirth is a method of delivering a baby without

the use of medications or interventions that might slow down or alter the natural progression of labor. Some women choose natural birth because it allows them to experience the process of childbirth without the potential side effects and risks associated with medications. Others may prefer the idea of natural birth for personal or cultural reasons.

## Advantages of Natural Birth:

1. Experience the Full Labor Process: Natural birth allows women to experience the full process of labor and delivery without any medication-induced interventions.

2. Fewer Medical Interventions: Natural birth eliminates the need for medical interventions such as epidurals, vacuum extraction, or forceps delivery, which might have potential medical risks and complications.

3. Shorter Recovery Time: Women who choose natural birth tend to have an easier recovery time than those who had medications or interventions during delivery.

## Disadvantages of Natural Birth:

1. Intense Pain: Natural birth can be extremely painful, and not all women can tolerate this without pain-relief medications.

2. Increased Stress and Anxiety: The pain associated with natural delivery can lead to increased stress levels and anxiety for the mother, which may affect the baby's well-being.

## Epidural:

An epidural is a procedure in which an anesthetic is injected into the epidural space in the lower part of the spinal cord, numbing the nerves that transmit pain signals from the uterus and cervix.

## Advantages of Epidural:

1. Pain Relief: Epidural injections provide women with significant pain relief, allowing them a more comfortable delivery process.

2. Less Stress and Anxiety: An epidural can help women feel more comfortable and relaxed during delivery, which can

reduce stress and anxiety levels.

## Disadvantages of Epidural:

1. Drowsiness and Nausea: Some women may feel drowsy or nauseous after receiving an epidural.

2. Increased Medical Intervention: Epidurals can lead to other medical interventions such as having additional delivery medication, getting a catheter, or needing interventions like vacuum extraction or forceps delivery.

3. Longer Labor Time: Women who receive epidural injections may encounter longer labor times than those who choose natural delivery.

In conclusion, the decision to go with natural birth or epidural depends on the level of comfort and individual preference. Women should discuss the pros and cons of both options with their healthcare provider and weigh up their personal benefits and risks of each option before making a decision.

# CHAPTER 5

## LABOR AND DELIVERY

### The stages of labor

There are three stages of labor:

First Stage:

The first stage of labor begins with the onset of true labor contractions that cause the cervix to dilate and efface, meaning it begins to thin out. This stage can be divided into two phases;

1. Early Labor Phase: This phase starts with the onset of labor through to when the cervix is around three to four centimeters dilated. During this phase, contractions usually last for 30 to 60 seconds, and they come at regular intervals of about 5 to 20 minutes. Women in early labor may feel anxious, excited, and nervous.

2. Active Labor Phase: This phase begins when the cervix is four centimeters or more dilated, and it progresses to full dilation, which is 10 centimeters. During this stage, contractions become more intense, longer, and closer together, with a duration of around 60 seconds, and coming at regular intervals of about 2 to 5 minutes. This phase can last between six to twelve hours.

**Second Stage:**

The second stage of labor is the pushing stage, which begins when the cervix is fully dilated and continues until the baby's birth. In this phase, the baby begins to move down the birthing canal, and the mother-in-law starts experiencing an urge to push. This stage can last between 20 minutes and up to two hours or more, depending on the position of the baby, the mother's strength and endurance, and other factors.

**Third Stage:**

The third stage of labor is the delivery of the placenta. After the baby's birth, the mother continues to experience contractions that help deliver the placenta. This stage can last between five to 30 minutes, and some women may need assistance from their healthcare provider to deliver the placenta.

Every woman experiences each stage of labor differently. Still, understanding the characteristics of each stage and the signs that labor is progressing, such as the onset of regular and more intense contractions, can help prepare for this process and make informed decisions. It's essential to have a healthcare provider's support throughout the labor and delivery process and communicate any concerns or changes in symptoms or progress experienced.

## Vaginal birth vs. Cesarean section

Vaginal birth and Cesarean section (C-section) are two delivery methods used to birth babies, with each having its advantages and disadvantages depending on the mother's and baby's health conditions and any potential complications.

**Vaginal Birth:**

Vaginal birth is a natural form of delivery in which the baby passes through the vagina or birth canal. This birth method is done with or without medical interventions, depending on the mother's preferences and the monitoring of the baby's well-being. Natural birth can occur spontaneously or through induced labor, and it is often quicker than a C-section. The advantages and disadvantages of vaginal birth include the following:

**Advantages:**

1. Shorter Recovery Time: Mothers who choose vaginal birth typically have a shorter recovery time than those who have C-sections.

2. Lower Complication Risks: Vaginal birth poses fewer risks of complications such as blood loss and infections.

3. Lower Respiratory Issues in the Baby: Babies born vaginally are less likely to have respiratory issues after birth.

**Disadvantages:**

1. Painful and Intense: Vaginal birth is naturally painful and can be an intense experience for women.

2. Potential Tears and Episiotomy: Women giving birth vaginally may experience tears in the perineum or need an episiotomy, a surgical cut made by the healthcare provider to widen the vaginal opening to prevent further tearing.

3. Newborn Head Trauma: In some cases, the baby's head can become misshaped or bruised during vaginal birth.

**Cesarean Section:**

A Cesarean section is a surgical delivery method in which the baby is delivered via an incision made in the mother's abdomen and uterus. C-sections are often chosen in cases of complications or when vaginal birth poses risks to the mother, baby, or both. The advantages and disadvantages of the Cesarean section include the following:

**Advantages:**

1. Planned Delivery: A C-section allows for the delivery date to be planned.

2. Avoids Labor and Birth Trauma: A C-section can avoid potential trauma experienced during labor and delivery, such as tears or episiotomies.

3. May Benefit High-Risk Pregnancies: C-sections can be beneficial for high-risk pregnancies and reduce the risks of complications for the mother and baby.

**Disadvantages:**

1. Risk of Infection: C-sections pose a higher risk of infection due to being a surgical procedure.

2. Longer Recovery Time: Mothers who undergo C-sections require a more extended recovery time than those who deliver vaginally due to the surgery.

3. Potential Breathing Issues in the Baby: C-section babies may experience respiratory issues after birth due to the lack of compression of the birth canal along with hormonal and breathing changes during labor.

Lastly, both vaginal birth and Cesarean section each have their advantages and drawbacks depending on the mother's and baby's health conditions and any potential complications. The choice of delivery method should be made after weighing the potential risks and benefits associated with each method. A healthcare provider's expert guidance can assist in making an informed decision that is best for the mother and baby's health.

## Labor pain management options

Labor is a painful experience for most women, but there are various pain management options available to help them cope. Some of the commonly used pain management options include:

1. Relaxation Techniques: Deep breathing, meditation, yoga, and visualization are popular relaxation techniques used to help manage labor pain. These techniques help distract women from the pain and promote a sense of calm and focus.

2. Hydrotherapy: Water births, showers, and baths are often recommended as natural pain relief options during labor. The warm water helps to soothe the body and alleviate the pain.

3. TENS (Transcutaneous Electrical Nerve Stimulators) Machine: A TENS machine is a small electronic device that sends electrical pulses through electrodes placed on the skin, blocking pain signals from reaching the brain. TENS machines do not interfere with labor hormones and can be used throughout labor.

4. Nitrous Oxide (Laughing Gas): Nitrous oxide is a gas that is inhaled through a mask. It provides temporary pain relief, reduces anxiety, and allows women to remain fully conscious and in control during labor.

5. Epidural: Epidural is the most commonly administered pain relief option during labor. It involves an injection of an anesthetic into the lower back, which numbs the lower half of the body, including the uterus and cervix. Epidurals provide

effective pain relief, allowing women to rest and conserve energy during labor.

6. Narcotics: Narcotic pain relievers such as fentanyl are effective in managing labor pain. They are usually administered through an IV and are most effective in the early stages of labor.

7. Acupuncture: Acupuncture is a traditional Chinese medicine practice that involves inserting thin needles into the skin. It stimulates the release of endorphins that help alleviate pain and promote relaxation during labor.

There are various pain management options available to women during labor. It's important to discuss and plan with a healthcare provider well ahead of delivery to choose the best option that aligns with personal preferences for a comfortable and safe labor experience.

## What happens after delivery

After delivery, a new chapter begins, and there are many things that happen to both the mother and the newborn. Here is a detailed explanation of what takes place after delivery:

1. Placenta Delivery: After a baby is born, the mother needs to deliver the placenta. The uterus continues to contract to push the placenta out, which typically occurs within 15 to 30 minutes of delivery.

2. Checking Vital Signs: After delivery, the healthcare provider checks the mother's vital signs such as blood pressure, temperature, and heart rate. These checks ensure that the mother is recovering well and that no complications have arisen.

3. Skin-to-Skin Contact: Immediate skin-to-skin contact between the mother and baby is encouraged shortly after birth to promote bonding, and breastfeeding, to regulate the baby's temperature.

4. Assessing and Cleaning the Baby: After being handed over, the healthcare provider assesses the baby's health and checks vital signs. The baby is cleaned and evaluated for any signs of distress.

5. Umbilical Cord Care: The umbilical cord is often clamped, and cut a few minutes after birth. The stump of the cord dries up and eventually falls off in one to two weeks.

6. Newborn Screening Tests: Screening for hearing loss, metabolic disorders, and other health conditions is typically

performed within the first few days of life.

7. Breastfeeding: Breastfeeding is typically initiated within the first hour after birth to ensure the baby receives the essential nutrients and to promote the development of the mother-baby bond.

8. Checking for Post-partum Complications: The healthcare provider checks the mother for post-partum complications, such as heavy bleeding, infection, and blood clots.

9. Post-partum Recovery and Discharge: After delivery, mothers may require hospital admission for a post-partum recovery period. Before discharge, healthcare providers conduct a thorough evaluation and assessment of the mother and baby to determine their health status. The discharge plan includes discussing proper post-partum care, warning signs, and follow-up appointments.

In summary, after delivery, the healthcare providers take several steps to ensure the mother and baby are healthy and recovering well. They monitor vital signs, c-section incisions or tears in the perineum, promote bonding, and discuss various post-delivery care requirements. Mothers and their families must maintain open communication with healthcare providers and attend follow-up appointments for a healthy recovery of both the mother and baby in the postnatal period.

# CHAPTER 6

## POSTPARTUM CARE

### Recovery after childbirth

Recovery after childbirth, also known as the postnatal period, is a critical time for both the mother and the newborn. Here is a detailed explanation of the recovery process after childbirth:

1. Physical Recovery: After childbirth, the body transitions from pregnancy to birth. Mothers may experience physical discomforts such as vaginal tenderness, abdominal pain, and breastfeeding pain. Over time, these discomforts should subside, and the mother's body should return to its pre-pregnancy state.

2. Emotional Recovery: Recovery from childbirth involves a range of emotional and psychological changes. The mother might experience feelings of exhaustion, anxiety, depression, and mood swings. The support of family, friends, and

healthcare providers can help her navigate these changes.

3. Postpartum Check-up: The mother should schedule a postpartum check-up with her healthcare provider a few weeks after delivery. The healthcare provider will assess the mother's physical and emotional recovery and offer advice on postpartum care.

4. Nutrition: Recovery after childbirth requires a nutritious diet that helps the mother recover physically and emotionally. A healthy diet rich in fruits, vegetables, whole grains, and lean protein, helps the body heal and regain strength and also promotes healthy breastfeeding for the baby.

5. Exercise: After delivery, mothers are encouraged to start gentle exercises as soon as they feel comfortable; walking, postnatal yoga, and gentle stretches are ideal. These exercises help to improve physical recovery, relieve stress, and boost energy.

6. Caring for the Baby: Recovering from childbirth involves caring for the newborn, which can be challenging for a new mother. Proper support from family, friends, and healthcare providers can help ease the process of caring for the newborn.

7. Rest: Rest is essential for recovery after childbirth. New mothers need rest to help their bodies heal and regain energy. New mothers are encouraged to sleep whenever possible and

limit activities that require too much energy or exertion.

Considering the physical, emotional, and socio-economic changes that follow childbirth, good self-care is vital for a new mother. Recovery after childbirth is a gradual process, and mothers should take the time to rest, eat well, exercise, and get the necessary emotional support from family, friends, or healthcare providers. Additionally, new mothers should attend post-partum check-ups for proper medical care and attention to ensure that they recover optimally.

## Breastfeeding and bottle-feeding

Breastfeeding and bottle-feeding are two ways of feeding a newborn, and each has its advantages and disadvantages. Here is a detailed discussion of breastfeeding and bottle-feeding:

**Breastfeeding:**

Breastfeeding is the recommended way to feed newborns as it provides essential nutrients, and antibodies, and promotes mother-baby bonding. Here are some of the benefits of breastfeeding:

1. Nutrition: Breast milk provides the perfect balance of nutrients that newborns need for growth and development.

2. Antibodies: Breast milk contains antibodies that protect the baby from infections and illnesses.

3. Saves money: Breast milk is free, and mothers can save a lot of money by not purchasing formula.

4. Convenience: Breastfeeding is very convenient as it requires no preparation, no sterilization, and is always available on demand.

5. Promotes bonding: Breastfeeding promotes a strong mother-baby bond, which benefits both the mother and the baby.

However, breastfeeding can be challenging for some mothers. Some of the challenges may include:

1. Pain: Breastfeeding can cause sore nipples and, in some cases, breastfeeding can cause infections.

2. Inconvenience: Breastfeeding can be inconvenient at times, especially if the mother needs to be away from the baby for long periods.

3. Misconceptions: There are many misconceptions about breastfeeding, which can make some new mothers feel intimidated or embarrassed to breastfeed.

**Bottle-feeding:**

Bottle feeding involves using formula or expressed breast milk to feed the newborn. Here are some of the advantages of bottle-feeding:

1. Control: Bottle feeding allows the parents to control the timing and amount of food the baby receives.

2. Convenience: Bottle feeding is convenient as other caregivers, such as fathers and grandparents, can also participate in the feeding.

3. Flexibility: Bottle feeding is very flexible, and mothers can choose to use formula or expressed milk and switch between the two without any issues.

However, bottle feeding also has some disadvantages. They include:

1. Cost: Formula can be expensive, and the cost can add up over time.

2. Preparation: Bottle-feeding requires preparation, such as sterilization of the bottles and making the formula.

3. Lack of antibodies: The formula does not provide the same antibodies as breast milk does, which makes the baby more susceptible to infections and illness.

Both breastfeeding and bottle-feeding have advantages and disadvantages. Ultimately the decision lies with the mother and what works best for her and the baby. New mothers should consult their healthcare provider for advice on feeding the baby and choose the feeding method that is the most beneficial for themselves and their newborn.

## Your newborn's health and well-being

As a parent, ensuring your newborn's health and well-being is a top priority. Here are some factors that can contribute to your newborn's health and well-being:

1. Nutrition: Providing your newborn with proper nutrition is essential for their health and well-being. Breastfeeding provides essential nutrients and antibodies that help fight off infections and build strong immune systems. If breastfeeding isn't possible, infant formula is the best alternative.

2. Immunization: Immunizations protect your newborn from diseases, infections, and illnesses, which is critical for their overall health and well-being. Consult with your healthcare provider to determine which vaccines are necessary.

3. Hygiene: Maintaining proper hygiene for your newborn is essential to prevent infections. You should wash your hands before handling your newborn and ensure your newborn's environment, such as changing tables, toys, and bedding, are clean and sanitized.

4. Sleep: Newborns require a lot of sleep, and proper sleep is necessary for their physical and mental development. Create a safe and comfortable sleep environment for the baby, and ensure they are placed on their backs to prevent sudden infant death syndrome (SIDS).

5. Physical activity: Although newborns do not need structured physical activity like adults, gently playing with your newborn can help them develop their muscles and coordination.

6. Medical checkups: Regular checkups with your healthcare provider can ensure that your newborn is meeting their developmental milestones and is healthy overall.

7. Emotional support: Newborns also need emotional support

and social interaction. Spend quality time with your newborn by smiling, talking to them, and cuddling them. This helps build strong emotional bonds and contributes to their overall well-being.

Remember, newborns are fragile and require a lot of care and attention. By providing proper nutrition, immunizing them, maintaining proper hygiene, ensuring they get adequate sleep and physical activity, going for regular medical checkups, and offering emotional support, you can ensure that your newborn is healthy and well.

## Coping with the emotional rollercoaster of motherhood

Motherhood can be a joyful and fulfilling experience, but it can also be an emotional rollercoaster. Here are some tips for coping with the emotional ups and downs of motherhood:

1. Accepting your emotions: The first step in coping with difficult emotions is to accept them. Understand that it is normal to feel a range of emotions, including joy, frustration, anxiety, and exhaustion.

2. Seeking support: Talking to a trusted friend, family member, or therapist can provide a safe outlet to share your feelings and

receive emotional support.

3. Self-care: Taking care of yourself is essential for your emotional well-being. This includes eating healthily, getting enough sleep, exercising, and engaging in hobbies or activities that bring you joy.

4. Prioritizing: Trying to do everything can add to your stress levels. Prioritize your tasks and delegate when possible. Remember that it is okay to say "no" to things that do not align with your priorities.

5. Adjusting your expectations: Motherhood can be challenging, and adjusting your expectations can help you cope with the emotional ups and downs. Be kind to yourself and recognize that you are doing the best you can.

6. Practicing mindfulness: Mindfulness can help you stay grounded and focus on the present moment. You can practice mindfulness through meditation, deep breathing, or yoga.

7. Connecting with your baby: Focus on the positive moments and take time to connect with your baby. This can help you feel more grounded and reduce feelings of stress and anxiety.

Remember, coping with the emotional rollercoaster of motherhood takes time and patience, and it is okay to ask for help. Be kind to yourself and prioritize your emotional well-being.

# CHAPTER 7

## POSTPARTUM DEPRESSION

### Symptoms and causes of postpartum depression

Postpartum depression (PPD) is a mood disorder that affects some women after childbirth. Symptoms and causes of PPD can vary from woman to woman, but here are some common factors:

Symptoms:

- Sadness or crying for no apparent reason

- Feelings of worthlessness, guilt, or hopelessness

- Irritability, anger, or agitation

- Difficulty bonding with the baby

- Changes in appetite or sleep patterns

- Fatigue or lack of energy

- Loss of interest in activities once enjoyed

Thoughts of harming oneself or their baby (rare but a serious symptom)

**Causes:**

- Hormonal changes: Hormonal changes during pregnancy and after childbirth can affect a woman's mood and emotional state.

- History of depression: Women with a history of depression or other mental health disorders may be at a higher risk for PPD.

- Life stressors: Stressful life events, such as financial difficulties or relationship problems, can increase the risk of PPD.

- Pregnancy or childbirth complications: Women who experience pregnancy or childbirth complications, such as premature birth or medical complications, may be more vulnerable to PPD.

- Lack of social support: Women with a lack of social support, such as a partner, family member, or friend, may be at a higher risk of PPD.

It is important to seek medical attention if you experience symptoms of PPD. Treatment options such as therapy, medication, or a combination of both can be effective in managing symptoms of PPD.

## How to prevent and treat postpartum depression

Preventing and treating postpartum depression (PPD) can involve a combination of self-care, lifestyle changes, and medical treatment. Here are some steps you can take to prevent or treat PPD:

1. Prioritize self-care: Take care of yourself physically and emotionally. Eat well, get enough sleep, exercise, and engage in activities that you enjoy.

2. Stay connected: Connect with others, such as friends, family, or a support group for new parents.

3. Seek help early: Don't hesitate to reach out to your healthcare provider if you experience symptoms of PPD. Early

intervention can help prevent symptoms from worsening.

4. Consider therapy: Therapy, such as cognitive-behavioral therapy (CBT), can be effective in treating PPD. It can help you identify negative thoughts and behaviors and develop healthier coping mechanisms.

5. Medication: Antidepressants may be prescribed to treat PPD. It is important to discuss any concerns or questions you may have with your healthcare provider.

6. Mind-body therapies: Mindfulness-based stress reduction (MBSR), yoga, or acupuncture may also be beneficial in managing PPD symptoms.

7. Involve your partner: Your partner can play an important role in supporting you during this time. Involve them in your care plan and communicate your needs with them.

Remember, PPD is a treatable condition, and with early intervention and appropriate care, you can recover. Don't hesitate to reach out for help if you need it and prioritize your self-care.

## Coping Strategies for new mothers

Coping strategies can be helpful for new mothers as they adjust to their new roles and deal with the challenges of motherhood. Here are some coping strategies that can be useful:

1. Take breaks: Giving yourself a break when you need it can help you recharge and reduce stress. Ask for help from family or friends, or consider hiring a babysitter for a few hours.

2. Practice self-care: Taking care of yourself physically and emotionally is important. Eat healthy, engage in regular exercise, and look for ways to relax and unwind, such as taking a warm bath or meditating.

3. Stay connected: Seek out the support of other new mothers through support groups or social networks. Sharing experiences can help you feel less isolated and provide a sense of community.

4. Manage stress: Identify the sources of stress in your life and find ways to manage them. This may include practicing relaxation techniques, such as deep breathing or visualization exercises.

5. Prioritize sleep: Sleep deprivation can make it difficult to cope with daily stressors. Try to get as much sleep as possible and take naps when you can.

6. Lower your expectations: It's easy to feel overwhelmed by the demands of motherhood. Try to set realistic expectations for yourself and your baby, and be gentle with yourself as you adjust to your new role.

7. Seek professional help: If you are struggling to cope or feel overwhelmed, don't hesitate to seek professional help. Your healthcare provider can provide guidance and support, or refer you to a mental health professional if needed.

Remember that adjusting to motherhood can take time, and it's important to take care of yourself as well as your child. By incorporating these coping strategies into your daily routine, you can better manage stress and enjoy the journey of motherhood.

# CHAPTER 8

## SPECIAL SITUATIONS

### High-risk pregnancies

A high-risk pregnancy is a pregnancy in which the mother or the baby is at an increased risk of complications during pregnancy, labor, delivery, or after delivery. Some factors that can increase the risk of a high-risk pregnancy include:

1. Maternal age: Women who are over the age of 35 are at an increased risk for complications.

2. Medical conditions: Women who have pre-existing medical conditions such as diabetes, hypertension, heart, or kidney disease are at increased risk.

3. Past pregnancy complications: Women who have had previous preterm births, stillbirths, or miscarriages are at increased risk.

4. Multiple pregnancies: Women carrying twins, triplets or more are more likely to experience complications.

5. Lifestyle factors: Smoking, alcohol, and drug use can increase the risk of complications.

6. Obesity: Women who are obese have an increased risk of complications during pregnancy.

7. Infections: Certain infections during pregnancy can increase the risk of complications, such as Zika, cytomegalovirus (CMV), and chickenpox.

High-risk pregnancies require specialized care and monitoring by a healthcare provider. Depending on the risk factor involved, additional tests and procedures may be recommended, such as more frequent prenatal visits, ultrasounds, or blood tests. If complications arise, early intervention and treatment are crucial to reduce the risk of adverse outcomes for both the mother and the baby.

It is important for women to attend regular prenatal care appointments, and to talk to a healthcare provider if they have any concerns about their pregnancy or feel like they may be at risk for a high-risk pregnancy. Being informed and proactive can help to minimize the risks and ensure the best possible outcomes for both mother and baby.

# Multiples

Multiples refer to a pregnancy in which a woman is expecting more than one baby at the same time. Twins are the most common type of multiple pregnancies, followed by triplets, quadruplets, and higher-order multiples. The occurrence of multiples in pregnancy can happen naturally as a result of the fertilization of more than one egg or through assisted reproductive technologies such as fertility treatments.

Pregnancies with multiples are considered high-risk pregnancies, which means they require careful monitoring and specialized medical care to ensure the health and well-being of both the mother and the babies. Some of the potential risks associated with multiples pregnancies may include:

1. Preterm labor and delivery: Women carrying multiples are at an increased risk of preterm labor and delivery, which puts the babies at risk for complications.

2. Low birth weight: Babies born as multiples may be smaller in size and have a lower birth weight, which increases their risk for certain health problems.

3. Preeclampsia: Women carrying multiples are at an increased risk of developing preeclampsia, a serious pregnancy

complication characterized by high blood pressure and protein in the urine.

4. Cesarean delivery: The likelihood of cesarean delivery is higher in multiple pregnancies due to the increased risk of complications during vaginal delivery.

5. Twin-to-twin transfusion syndrome (TTTS): This is a rare but serious condition that can occur in identical twin pregnancies where one twin receives more blood than the other.

Management of a multiple pregnancy involves early and regular prenatal care, careful monitoring of the mother and babies, and possible interventions to reduce the risk of complications. The healthcare provider may also recommend lifestyle changes such as rest, nutrition, and hydration, as well as certain medications to support a healthy pregnancy. By working closely with their healthcare provider and following their recommendations, women with multiples can increase their chances of a safe and healthy pregnancy.

## Pregnancy after infertility

Pregnancy after infertility refers to a pregnancy that occurs after a woman has experienced difficulty getting pregnant, such as with infertility or fertility treatments. This can be a very emotional time for women who have struggled to conceive, and there may be additional physical and emotional concerns that come with this type of pregnancy.

On one hand, pregnancy after infertility can be a source of great joy and relief after months or years of trying to conceive. However, it can also be a time of anxiety and worry, particularly during the early stages of pregnancy, due to the fear of miscarriage or other complications.

To support a healthy pregnancy after infertility, it is important to maintain regular prenatal care and to work closely with a healthcare provider to monitor the pregnancy. Depending on the individual circumstances, additional testing and monitoring may be recommended to ensure the health of both the mother and the baby.

Women who are pregnant after infertility may also benefit from supportive care, such as counseling or support groups, to help manage any emotional concerns. It is normal to experience a wide range of emotions during pregnancy after infertility, and seeking out support can be helpful in navigating any challenges that may arise.

Overall, with proper care and support, women can go on to have healthy and successful pregnancies after infertility. It is important to stay positive and focused on staying healthy throughout the pregnancy, while also taking time to address any emotional concerns that may arise.

## Pregnancy after a loss

Pregnancy after a loss refers to a pregnancy that occurs after a miscarriage, stillbirth, or neonatal death. This can be a very emotional time for women and their partners, and there may be additional physical and emotional concerns that come with this type of pregnancy.

On one hand, pregnancy after a loss can be a source of hope and healing, providing an opportunity to start again and move forward. However, it can also be a time of anxiety and fear, particularly during the early stages of pregnancy, due to the fear of another loss.

To support a healthy pregnancy after a loss, it is important to maintain regular prenatal care and to work closely with a healthcare provider to monitor the pregnancy. Depending on the individual circumstances, additional testing and monitoring may be recommended to ensure the health of both the mother and the baby.

Women who are pregnant after a loss may also benefit from

supportive care, such as counseling or support groups, to help manage any emotional concerns. It is normal to experience a wide range of emotions during a pregnancy after a loss, and seeking out support can be helpful in navigating any challenges that may arise.

Overall, with proper care and support, women can go on to have healthy and successful pregnancies after a loss. It is important to stay positive and focused on staying healthy throughout the pregnancy, while also taking time to address any emotional concerns that may arise.

# CHAPTER 9

## YOUR NEW FAMILY

### Adjusting to life as a new mother

Adjusting to life as a new mother can be both exciting and challenging. It is a time of significant change as you learn to care for your newborn, establish new routines, and adapt to the demands of motherhood. Here are some tips for adjusting to life as a new mother:

1. Take it one day at a time: It is important to focus on the present moment and not get too caught up in worrying about the future. Try to enjoy the baby and cherish each moment.

2. Get support: Reach out to friends, family, and professionals for help and support. You can join mother groups or reach out to other new mothers facing the same issues.

3. Get some rest: Try to get as much rest as possible, sleep

when the baby sleeps, and take naps whenever you can. Rest is crucial to help you recharge and give you the energy you need to care for your baby.

4. Ask for help: Don't be afraid to ask for help whenever you need it. It is impossible to do everything on your own, so ask your partner, family members, or friends for help when you need it.

5. Be kind to yourself: Remember, it is normal to make mistakes, and you will learn as you go. Give yourself permission to make mistakes and be kind to yourself.

6. Connect with other new mothers: Join a mother's group or attend a baby-friendly activity. Socializing with other mothers can help you feel connected and supported during what can be a lonely time.

Remember, every mother's experience is different, and there is no right or wrong way to adjust to life as a new mother. The most important thing is to focus on taking care of yourself and your baby and to seek support whenever you need it.

# Balancing work and family

Balancing work and family can be a challenging task, as it requires careful planning and prioritizing. Here are some tips for achieving a balanced work-life balance:

1. Set clear boundaries: It is essential to create clear boundaries between your work and home life. This means scheduling specific times for work, and specific times for family and personal activities.

2. Communicate with your employer: Discuss your work-life balance needs with your employer. If possible, try to negotiate flexible work arrangements such as flexible hours, working from home, or job-sharing.

3. Create a schedule: Plan out your week to ensure that you have enough time for work, family, and personal activities. Incorporate family time into your schedule and prioritize important activities.

4. Outsource tasks: Consider delegating some tasks to others, such as hiring a cleaning service or ordering groceries online. This will help free up time for more important activities.

5. Take time for self-care: Make sure to take time for self-care

activities such as exercise, hobbies, or meditation. Taking care of yourself will help you maintain a healthy work-life balance.

6. Be present: When you are at home, try to be fully present with your family and avoid distractions such as emails or work-related tasks.

Remember, achieving a balanced work-life balance is an ongoing process, and it requires flexibility, open communication, and a willingness to make adjustments when necessary. By setting clear boundaries, communicating with your employer, strategizing, outsourcing, taking time for self-care, and being present, you can create a healthy balance between your work and family life.

## Nurture and care for your new family

Nurturing and caring for a new family requires attention, patience, and dedication. Here are some tips to help you in this process:

1. Establish a routine: Creating a daily routine can help your family establish structure and consistency. This can include setting a regular bedtime, mealtimes, and designated playtime.

2. Prioritize self-care: Taking care of yourself is an important aspect of nurturing your family. This includes getting enough sleep, eating healthy meals, staying physically active, and taking breaks when needed.

3. Communicate openly: Good communication is essential in any relationship, and it is especially important in a new family. Make sure to communicate openly and honestly with your partner and children to ensure that everyone's needs are being met.

4. Be present: Being present at the moment will help you connect with your family and build strong relationships. Try to minimize distractions, such as phones or emails, during family time.

5. Embrace traditions: Developing family traditions is a great way to create memories and build a sense of togetherness. This can include holiday celebrations, family game nights, or weekly dinners.

6. Practice forgiveness and grace: No family is perfect, and mistakes will inevitably happen. Practice forgiving and grace towards one another to create a supportive and loving environment.

Remember, nurturing and caring for your new family is a

process that requires patience and effort. By establishing a routine, prioritizing self-care, communicating openly, being present, embracing traditions, and practicing forgiveness and grace, you can build strong family relationships and create a loving environment for your new family.

# CONCLUSION

## Your new journey as a mother

Becoming a mother marks the start of a new journey, one filled with joy, love, and challenges. As you navigate this new path, here are some tips to help you along the way:

1. Practice Self-care: Remember to take care of yourself, both physically and mentally. This means getting enough sleep, eating healthy foods, staying physically active, and taking breaks when needed.

2. Be present: Being present at the moment will help you build strong connections with your child. Put away distractions such as phones or computers during feeding and playtime.

3. Take it slow: You and your baby are both learning and adjusting to this new life. Give yourself time to learn and take it one day at a time.

4. Ask for help: Don't be afraid to ask for help from family or friends. It's okay to lean on others during this transition.

5. Bond with your baby: Bonding with your baby is essential for their emotional and physical development. Spend time talking, singing, and playing with your baby to strengthen the bond.

6. Find support: Join a new parent support group, talk to other moms, or seek professional support. Surround yourself with people who can offer guidance, support, and advice.

Remember, each mother's journey is unique. Be patient with yourself and your baby and take time to savor these special moments as you begin this new chapter in your life.

## Enjoying the experience of pregnancy and new motherhood

In conclusion, pregnancy and motherhood are experiences unlike any other. Despite the numerous challenges that come with them, they can also be sources of profound joy and fulfillment. By embracing the ups and downs of this journey, you can come to appreciate the incredible strength and resilience that you possess, both as a mother and as a person.

While each person's experiences are unique, there are certain things that can help make this time more enjoyable. These include taking care of yourself, both physically and mentally, surrounding yourself with supportive people, and finding ways to appreciate the little things in life.

Whether it's the sensation of your baby's first kicks or the sound of their first giggles, being present and savoring these moments can help you connect more deeply with your child and create lasting memories.

So, to all the expectant and new mothers out there, know that your journey is worth it and that the love and joy that you will experience through it all is immeasurable. Embrace the challenges, find support, and enjoy the experience of pregnancy and new motherhood. It will be a ride that you'll never forget.

## Tips for managing the challenges and cherishing the joys of motherhood

Motherhood can be wonderful, but it also comes with its own unique set of challenges. Here are some tips for managing these challenges while cherishing the joys of motherhood:

1. Accept help from family and friends: There is no shame in accepting help from others, especially during those first few

months when you are adjusting to being a new mom.

2. Make time for yourself: This is important for your mental health. Schedule some time, even just a few minutes, every day to do something that you enjoy.

3. Connect with other moms: Join a moms group or take part in activities where you can chat with other moms. This can help you feel less alone and more supported.

4. Prioritize sleep: Sleep is vital to your physical and mental health. Do your best to get quality sleep whenever possible.

5. Get outside: Fresh air and sunshine can do wonders for your mood. Try to get outside for a walk or some other activity every day.

6. Focus on the positive: It can be easy to get bogged down in the challenges of motherhood. Make a conscious effort to focus on the positive moments and savor them.

7. Cherish the small moments: Snuggles, first smiles, and giggles are all milestones that are easy to miss if you're not paying attention. Take the time to notice and savor these small moments.

In short, motherhood is a journey full of both joys and

challenges. By being kind to yourself, accepting help, and finding ways to connect with both your child and other moms, you can navigate the challenges while cherishing the joys of motherhood.

## Taking pleasure in the experience of pregnancy and becoming a new mother

In conclusion, becoming pregnant and being a mother are experiences that cannot be compared to anything else. In spite of the myriad of difficulties that are inextricably linked to them, they have the potential to be wellsprings of tremendous joy and fulfillment. You may grow to appreciate the great strength and resiliency that you possess, both as a mother and as a person, by embracing the ups and downs of this journey. This is true for both you and your child.

There are some things that, despite the fact that everyone's experiences are different, may assist to make this time that much more joyful. Taking care of yourself, both physically and emotionally, surrounding yourself with people who are helpful, and finding ways to appreciate the little things in life are some of the things that fall under this category.

It does not matter if it is the feeling of your baby's first kicks or the sound of their first chuckles; being present and appreciating these moments may help you connect with your kid on a deeper level and build memories that will last a lifetime.

Know that your journey will be worth it and that the love and pleasure that you will experience through it all will be unmeasurable. This message goes out to all of the women who are now expecting or who have already given birth. Embrace the difficulties, surround yourself with people who can provide you with support, and make the most of the experience of being pregnant and a new mother. You will not soon forget the trip that lies ahead of you.

Advice for dealing with the difficulties of parenting while still appreciating its many blessings

The experience of motherhood can be rewarding, but it also comes with its own particular set of difficulties. Here are some suggestions for overcoming these obstacles while still taking pleasure in the many blessings of motherhood:

1. Do not feel guilty about receiving assistance from loved ones and close friends. This is especially important during the first few months of motherhood when you are still getting used to your new role as a parent.

2. Dedicate some time to oneself; doing so is essential for maintaining good mental health. Set aside some time every day, even if it is just a few minutes, to engage in an activity that brings you pleasure.

3. Establish connections with other mothers by participating in activities or joining a group for mothers where you will be able to talk to other mothers. You could feel less isolated and more supported as a result of this.

4. Make getting enough sleep a top priority. Sleep is important for both your physical and mental well-being. Make it a priority to obtain plenty of restful sleep whenever you can.

5. Get some exercise and some fresh air. Sunlight and clean air have been shown to have a positive effect on mood. Make it a point to go for a walk or engage in some other form of physical activity every single day.

6. Keep an optimistic outlook: It is easy to become mired down in the difficulties of parenting, thus it is important to keep an optimistic outlook. Put some effort into concentrating on the good parts of the experience and taking pleasure in them.

7. Take pleasure in the little things: Snuggles, first grins, and laughter are all significant moments that may easily be missed if one is not paying attention to what is going on around them.

Spend some time focusing on and appreciating the little things that happen during the day.

In a nutshell, becoming a mother is a journey that is filled with both joys and hardships. You are able to negotiate the obstacles of motherhood while still cherishing the joys of parenthood if you are nice to yourself if you are willing to accept support, and if you find ways to connect with both your kid and other mothers.

As an author, I believe that feedback from my readers is crucial in improving my writing and providing a better experience for future readers. Therefore, I would like to request sincere feedback from those who have read this book.

I would appreciate it if you could share your honest thoughts and opinions about the book. What did you like about it? What could I have done better? Did it provide new insights? Did it help you in any way?

Your honest feedback will help me improve and provide an even better experience for readers in the future. Please feel free to share your opinions, suggestions, and criticisms.

Thank you for taking the time to read and provide your feedback. Your support and input are invaluable, and I look forward to hearing from you.